THREE WEEKS IN AFRICA

THE MISSIONAL WORK OF HOSPICE

Chaplain Donna Kasik

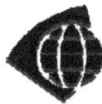

GlobalEdAdvance
Press

THREE WEEKS IN AFRICA

Copyright © 2012 by Donna Kasik

Library of Congress Control Number: 2012953773

Kasik, Donna 1961—

Three Weeks in Africa

ISBN 978-1-935434-13-9

Subject Codes and Description: 1. REL: 045000: Religion: Christian Ministry – Missions; 2. MED:042000 Medical: Terminal Care; 3. MED:011000: Medical: Caregiving.

Printed in Australia, Brazil, France, Germany, Italy, Spain, UK, and USA.

Book Cover Design by Brian Lane Green

Published by:

GlobalEdAdvance Press

a division of

Global Educational Advance, Inc.

Dedication:

To my new friends in Ndola, Zambia,

and to

All people involved in compassionate
End of life care.

Table of Contents

*"Life is stronger than death and
love is stronger than fear."*

Henri Nouwen

Foreword

Hospice care is considered to be the model for quality, compassionate care at the end of life, and involves a team-oriented approach of expert medical care, pain management, and emotional and spiritual support. These areas of concern are expressly tailored to the patient's needs and wishes. Emotional and spiritual support also is extended to the family and loved ones. Generally, this care is provided in the patient's home or in a home-like setting operated by a hospice program, and even within nursing homes and hospitals.

Many hospice care programs added palliative care to their names to reflect the range of care and services they provide, as hospice care and palliative care share the same core values and philosophies. Defined by the World Health Organization in 1990, palliative care seeks to address not only physical pain, but also emotional, social, and spiritual pain to achieve the best possible end of life care for patients and their families. Palliative care extends the principles of hospice care to a broader population that could benefit from receiving this type of care earlier in their illness or disease process. To better serve individuals who have advanced illness or are terminally ill, and their families, many hospice programs encourage access to care earlier in the illness or disease process. Health care professionals, who specialize in hospice and palliative care, work closely with staff and volunteers to address all the symptoms of illness, with the aim of promoting both comfort and dignity.

Since hospice and palliative care involves decisive care and compassion at a crucial time near the end of a person's life, why are faith-based groups not more involved in a missional way? In Africa, many of the hospices are founded by various churches and have a faith-based orientation. The American hospices are secular organizations that usually, though not always, incorporate spiritual care through trained, educated, ordained chaplains. The American hospice concept can appear to be more of a medical and social model and less spiritual than the faith-based groups that sponsor end of life care.

As a chaplain, who is a Christian, serving in hospice care, I believe the end of life has an extremely important spiritual component. As one faces the thoughts, questions, and beliefs of what might come after this life, individual's need spiritual guidance. Living on the threshold of eternity, the idea of an afterlife, coming to terms with one's mortality, the nature and existence of God, one's own life review, dealing with regrets and past mistakes and sins, which might include forgiveness extended towards others, as well as to oneself, requires the loving care of a spiritual counselor. Emotions might include depression, guilt, fear, or anger, and a person's spirituality and theology can either help or hinder their ability to process these often intense feelings. Can you imagine a more important time to come along side someone in a "missional" context, which means having a focus or "mission" based on one's faith? Yet there appears to be few people who view hospice or end of life care in a missional context, and few missionaries are involved in this type of ministry.

I was privileged to go to Ndola, Zambia to meet the hospice staff in that area and to learn how hospice and palliative care work is done is that country. Hospice and Palliative Care is a new concept in Africa, and is established, funded and carried out in different ways than American hospices. It was a blessing to be a part of this African journey and to share with others. My prayer is that this book will enable the reader to:

- Approach hospice care from a missional point of view,
- Share the importance of compassionate, faith-based end-of-life care, and
- Understand and appreciate Zambia's challenges of hospice and palliative care.

I would like to give credit to my friend, Dr. Paul Junker, who gave me the idea of writing this book. When I told him I would soon spend three weeks in Zambia, his reply was, "That sounds like the name of a book." Thus birthed the idea and name of this book: *Three Weeks in Africa – The Missional Work of Hospice.*

That's what true hospitality is all about, to offer a safe place, where the stranger can become a friend.

Henri Nouwen

*There is a yearning for love, unity, and communion
that doesn't go away.*

Henri Nouwen

Chapter One

Preparing for Africa

If you are a hospice worker, you already realize the many things that need to be done before you can get away for two or three weeks: patients need to be seen, charting needs to be completed, plans need to be made for patients in your absence, and all of the details that go along with hospice work. If you work in any other type of service or ministry work, you will also have many things to accomplish before leaving the country, and provisions to be made for work in your absence. But there are also many other items you need to check off your list before you can travel to Africa which you may have not even thought about:

- Inform your African hospice of your desire to visit.
- Go to a Travel Clinic.
- Have your Passport – make sure it is valid for more than six months after your return to the United States.
- Check on dates for travel.
- Plan your travel itinerary; purchase your plane ticket.

- Apply for your Visa.
- Purchase sun screen and insect repel-
  lant.
- Study the culture of the country you
  plan to visit.
- Pack.
- Plan to bring supplies and gifts.

These ten items listed above are the basic
necessities for your travel to your African hospice, and I have listed them in the order for
which it is easiest to accomplish.

**1. It is helpful to develop a relationship
prior to your arrival**, which will make for
a much more enjoyable and profitable visit.
Inform your African hospice of your desire to
travel to meet them, in order to deepen the
relationship and to assess the needs for a
more beneficial partnership. Ask them if there
is a particular time that is best for them for
you to visit, and inform them of a time that is
conducive to you. Share your enthusiasm to
visit and your desire to meet them for mutual
learning and benefit.

Hopefully, you have been in communication with your new friends from your African
hospice and have established a relationship
with them. I was in email communication with
the Zambian hospice manager for more than a
year, about once or twice a month. Our committee meets monthly as needed, or bi-month-

ly to discuss ideas for fundraising and to discern how to best partner with the Zambian hospice. I mail to Zambia the advertisements and brochures for our various fundraising activities so they can see what ideas we develop in order to accomplish this task. We want them to share in what we are doing to help bring local community and church awareness of the need to assist African countries with end of life care. Each member of our committee also emailed a message of introduction to help establish a relationship. Internet service is often difficult in many African countries, so do not be discouraged if you do not get a response, or if the response takes a long time to reach you.

2. I highly recommend making an appointment at your nearest Travel Clinic. These clinics are wonderful places, filled with all of the knowledge you will need concerning your particular African country. The clinic will inform you of any immunizations required, and how long in advance you will need to get them. Depending on what immunizations you will need, the dates of your travel may vary.

For example, if you need to be immunized for Hepatitis A & B, you will need to be immunized about <u>six months in advance</u>, since there is a three part series of shots you need to take over the span of about six months.

Also, you will need a yellow fever vaccine, which needs to be given at a minimum of ten days prior to travel. If you already have these immunizations, be sure to check the dates, since the yellow fever vaccine is only good for ten years, and may need to be updated. For instance, when I was in South Africa, making my connection to Zambia, in order to board the plane for Zambia, I needed to show proof of my yellow fever vaccine. These vaccines are very important, for your own health, as well as for your ability to enter the country.

The Travel Clinics will also give you valuable information about your particular African country concerning safety/crime, weather, and they will help give you an overall picture of your respective country. The clinic may frighten you if you have never been out of the country, especially when they tell you what precautions you need to take; they are simply doing their jobs, but a little common sense goes a long way. Don't worry; you will be fine.

You will also need to get a prescription for an anti-malaria medication, which they can give you and will explain how to take. I recommend taking a bottle of acidophilus along, since you will be taking an antibiotic for at least a month; the acidophilus helps your system during that time. The Travel Clinic will give you their recommendations and suggestions as well.

You will also be told not to drink the water – not to even brush your teeth with tap water, so be prepared to buy plenty of bottled water, and pack a few extra tooth brushes in case you forget and run your toothbrush under the sink water. It is a good idea to take chewable Pepto Bismal in case you have travelers' diarrhea.

3. Do you have a Passport that will still be valid six months after you plan to arrive home? If not, you will need to renew it. If you have never traveled abroad and do not have a Passport, you can go to your local Post Office, and they will help you obtain one. Make sure you begin the process of getting your Passport months before you even consider traveling.

4. There are important variables for scheduling travel dates: During certain times of the year it is less expensive to fly to certain African countries, which might be a priority for travel when considering your budget. Also, there are certain months when it is especially hot and dry or rainy in Africa, which might also be a consideration. Some months you will be more susceptible to mosquitoes, which carry malaria as well, so there are several variables you may want to consider. You should also consider the needs of your hospice or place of ministry where you work, such as their business during the holidays, etc. and when it is easiest on your team members for you to be away. You then need to determine how long you will be gone and request official vacation or leave for the trip.

5. Consider your travel itinerary once you have a valid Passport and received a response from your African partner concerning your travel:

- When do you want to leave?
- How long will you stay?
- Where all do you want to go in the country?
- How much time will you need before returning to work once you arrive back in America?

It is more convenient to leave on a Sunday because you have the previous week to complete your work and a whole Saturday for last minute details. Traveling to Africa, you may arrive two days later with the change in time zones. I booked my return flight for a Thursday, landing in America on Friday, which gave me the weekend to unpack and recover from jet lag (which you will indeed have!), and I returned to work Monday. Whatever schedule seems best for you is how you need to plan; mine is simply a suggestion.

Prices for flights vary tremendously, so be sure to check all possible carriers, or ask a travel agent to assist. I recommend purchasing the travel insurance since anything can happen that might force a change, and the airfare is quite expensive. I also strongly suggest taking a few days to "vacation" before leaving the country, since the travel is long and expensive, and you will need a few days to unwind from the experiences you will have at the hospice. Since the hospice I visited is in Zambia, I took a few days to travel to Livingstone and see Victoria Falls. I chose to take a coach bus there (which took twelve hours and only cost $33), which allowed me to see much of Zambia since Livingstone is on the opposite end of the country from Ndola.

There are usually safe, reliable buses that run to tourist locations, and they are much more affordable than small planes. I do not recommend any other form of public transportation, other than the coach buses, since many of the public transportation vehicles are unsafe and unreliable. Most African countries will offer safaris to see the animals; I strongly suggest taking advantage of this amazing opportunity if you have the funds.

6. Apply for your Visa once your plane ticket is purchased. Each country has specific requirements for Visas, so you need to do some research well in advance. The Internet makes obtaining a Visa quite simple; simply use whatever search engine you are comfortable with, type in "obtaining a Visa" for the country you will travel to, and follow the directions. The Embassy for the African country you will travel to is in Washington

D.C., and there is a phone number and an
email address if you need additional help. You
will need to have your itinerary and dates of
travel prior to applying for your Visa, which
is another reason to purchase the travel
insurance. For a minor technical reason, my
Visa was at first denied, but it was only a very
short time until the matter was taken care
of and my Visa arrived. Your Visa will cost
around $50 - $100, depending on the country.

**7. Make sure to purchase sunscreen
and insect repellant.** The sun is often very
hot and direct in Africa, and if you are fair
complexioned or have sensitive skin, you
will need sunscreen. Also, the antibiotic you
will be taking to prevent malaria will warn
you to avoid direct sunlight, which might not
always be possible. Purchase a good quality
sunscreen of at least 30 SPF (Sun-Protection
Factor), since you may be outside walking in
the sun with your African hospice workers.
Also, since malaria is prevalent in many
African countries, buy a good insect repellant
that repels mosquitoes in specific, with at
least 40% Deet. Your Travel Clinic can help
you with these items as well.

**8. If you have never been to Africa,
I highly suggest doing some research** in
advance to prevent embarrassment and
cultural insensitivity or blunders. There are
customs and greetings that will be unfamiliar
to you, so take the extra time to gather

information, which again is accessible on the Internet. You might also want to go to the Travel section of your local bookstore and buy a book on your African country.

For example, women in many African countries do not wear pants (in rural areas), but only dresses or skirts that come at least to the knee or below. Only children wear shorts; men do not. Women usually dress modestly, and generally do not wear tight-fitting clothing or anything revealing. Don't forget, you are representing your hospice, your church, or your mission board, as well as your country; dress appropriately.

Clothing is more relaxed in tourist areas, so if you opt for a safari or a tourist destination, you can wear pants, jeans, and even shorts.

9. Allow plenty of time to pack. Check with your airline how many pieces of luggage you can carry, what the maximum weight allowance is, and the cost of any additional luggage. Many airlines now allow only one bag of 50 pounds, with an additional fee of $60 to $75 for additional luggage. You are usually allowed one carry-on, and an additional purse, but again, within a certain size. If you are unsure, you can call the airline, or check online, and they will answer your questions. Make sure you pack a few lightweight long sleeve shirts/blouses, skirts, lightweight dresses, maybe a hat for the sun, closed-toe shoes, sandals, flip-flops, and comfortable walking shoes. If you are traveling during the rainy season, be sure to pack rain-gear. Do not bring your best clothes; look clean and respectable, but not wealthy. Do not make yourself a target for thieves.

I also recommend that you do not wear jewelry, or at least wear a minimum. Again, you do not want to draw attention to yourself or appear wealthy, and you want to appear more approachable to your partners at the hospice. Comfortable, casual skirts, tops, and dresses are best for women, and light-weight slacks and shirts for men. Use common sense.

10. I suggest saving one suitcase to bring your hospice some needed supplies. Supplies are expensive to ship to Africa from America. Again, good communication prior to your visit will ensure that you take the items they most need. When bringing protective gloves, it is best if you take them out of the box and put them in plastic bags for more space in your luggage. I brought various sizes of latex gloves, shoe and head protection, masks, disposable gowns and aprons, T-shirts from our 5K run fund-raiser (which they loved!), stethoscopes, gauze bandages, band aids, toothbrushes, and various training materials and information about hospice and palliative care, since these are relatively new concepts in Africa.

When considering what supplies to bring, remember that many of the patients will be HIV positive, so consider your personal safety, as well as the African hospice staff. Whatever you can afford to bring with you will be most appreciated.

***

FYI: Make copies of your Passport, just in case you lose yours or it is stolen; this probably will never happen, but photo copy your Passport just in case, and carry the copies in areas other than where you carry your Passport. It is a good idea to leave behind a copy of your Passport with your hospice, church, and/or family.

Are there people who keep telling each other the stories of hope and, together, go out and care for their fellow human beings, not pretending to solve all problems, but to bring a smile to a dying man and a little hope to a lonely child?

Henri Nouwen

Chapter Two

Handling Culture Shock:

A Field Guide

Surroundings

After many hours, probably days of travel, you will finally arrive at your destination. Hopefully, you contacted your partner hospice and they are waiting to greet you. The airport may be small and hot, with little organization. Since most people cannot afford cars, you will see many people walking, which will make roads, villages, and market places appear quite crowded. Many of the streets are mud, with huge potholes that fill up with water when it rains.

If you are fair complected, you may be stared at since there are few white people in many African countries, especially in rural areas. Again, do nothing to draw even more attention to yourself. If you carry a purse or backpack, hold onto it when you are in town or walking anywhere, though I suggest you only walk with your African friends from the hospice since they will look after you and know where you should and should not walk. I find it safe and comfortable to walk around in the daylight (never at night) with friends, for this allows you to take advantage of the many things you will experience in the countryside and around town.

You will see street markets made of sticks, mud and rags. I suggest you do not buy any food from these markets, but ask to be driven to the stores in town for your drinking water and any supplies or food you may need.

Poverty

Probably the most difficult adjustment in many countries in Africa is the extreme poverty. If you have never traveled to a Third World country, you will be shocked. I went with the hospice nurse and the caregivers (nurse aids) to the homes of their patients, which was emotionally draining. We visited one of the compounds which consisted of all mud huts and mud roads. Going from house to house, we sat in the dark unless the door was left open to allow in some sunlight. There were no windows, but there were soft chairs and usually a couch. The walls and floors were mud, and most of the homes had metal roofs secured to the walls only by large stones to weigh the roofs onto the walls of the houses.

The "kitchens" were small areas outside where food was prepared over an open fire of wood or charcoal. The "toilets" were pits dug outside of the house, with the appearance of a mud outhouse. The "bathroom," where people bathe, was a small plastic and stick enclosure. There was a common water pump at the front of the compound where people would carry their buckets, fill them with water, and carry back to their mud hut to bathe, cook, drink, and wash clothes. Most of our patients were HIV positive, and many were young widows. It is quite emotionally challenging.

Time

Time is very different in Africa. If someone says they will "pick you" (pick you up) at 8:00, they probably will not show up until at least 8:30; don't worry. There is also much less organization, and little structure relative to America. For example, I was told less than a week before I was to travel to Zambia that I would be part of a three-day teaching seminar on Hospice and Palliative Care at the local hospital. I was given a vague description of what they wanted me to speak about, but I had no idea about the timeframe, and to whom I would be speaking. I gathered together more than enough materials, and it was not until the day before the seminar that I was told how long I was expected to speak and who the audience would be.

The morning of the seminar, which was supposed to start at 8:30 a.m., my driver (yes, you will have a driver – you will never drive), picked me up at 8:30, made a few stops along the way, and dropped me off at the hospital at 9:45 for the 8:30 seminar! When I got to the room where I would be teaching (along with two other Zambians), one woman was there. Thirty people were supposed to attend, but their letter of invitation never reached them, there was no follow-up or confirmation, so the group of thirty nurses who were supposed to come was not there! The woman in charge of this training seminar started to make phone calls to invite student nurses to come; her third phone call was successful, and we would wait an hour for this group of student nurses to arrive.

When this woman was asked if she was upset or frustrated, she looked at me as if I had asked a strange question, and said, "No, why?" Such is life in Africa. No one is in a hurry in Africa, so be patient, and learn to wait – often. Life in Africa is a good exercise in developing patience. It is great that Luke wrote (21:19) "in your patience you gain souls." That is certainly needed in missional hospice and end of life care.

Structure

Since Africa is much more relaxed and far less structured than America, keep in mind that many of the rules and regulations we have at our hospices do not apply at all in Africa. Africans have a far different sense of time than Americans, so you might spend just a few minutes with one patient, but several hours with another. You may only see ten patients all week – depending on patient needs and hospice transportation. You will not have a productivity quota. A meeting may last half a day, while drinking tea together and sharing stories. The nurses and caregivers traveling to the patient's homes carried a notebook and a pen, and wrote a few notes – that was all of the documentation they did. Most of the visit was talking and counseling the patient, mostly about HIV and taking their medications properly.

Poor African hospices do not use computers in their work, so it is probably best to not even mention your laptop. Also, they do not have any initial assessment forms and visit forms that American hospices use, but I did share the basic patient information that we use, which can be tailored to their culture if they so choose. The Zambian hospice liked the idea of our "Care Plans," though they said they would need to adjust them to fit their culture. None of the hospice workers where I worked had vehicles, so the hospice driver picked them up along the way or at the office. Some workers took public transportation to the office, then were driven to a village where they walked from hut to hut. At the end of the day, the nurse called the driver on her cell phone to come back. Your daily routine will be much different than it is at home in America.

Children

By age three or four, many African children are running around by themselves, and few people seem to think anything about it; somehow, the children generally remain safe. You will, however, see many street children and orphans, which will break your heart. Be prepared. If you are fair skinned, many children might want to touch you and hear you speak, so enjoy them and grant them their wishes. Many children will be begging, and visitors are advised not to give them anything, but that is up to you. Just try to prepare yourself emotionally.

Lodging

Most guest houses are made of concrete, and are very simple, which is where you might stay. Depending on how long you are staying, you will probably wash your clothes each morning in a small washtub and hang them out to dry. In the evening when you return from your work, you will bring them in; allow more time for yourself than usual in the mornings for this purpose. You will not find a laundry mat in Africa, nor will you find a washer and dryer if you are in a rural area. Bring a pair of rubber sandals or flip-flops for walking around the house on the concrete floors, and for getting out of the shower or bathtub.

My guesthouse did not have a shower, but
I did have a clean bathtub that usually had
hot water, though occasionally the water was
out for a while. Keep a bucket of water in the
house for emergencies. Conserve your water; it
is quite valuable.

You will also see small lizards on the walls
of your house – not many – one or two. You
want them in your home to eat the mosquitoes or any other bugs, so **do not try to get
rid of them!** You will want to sleep under
your mosquito net each night, and tie it up
each morning.

The power often goes out in rural Africa,
and some places have "power sharing," where
your communities' power will be shut off for
several hours to give power to another community. Bring a flashlight for the times when
you will lose power and there are usually
candles and matches supplied in guest houses
for these times.

Many Africans are extremely clean, and
sweep and mop their homes daily, which you
might be expected to do if staying at a guesthouse. All homes and schools are in "compounds" which are enclosed, gated areas.
There is a gatekeeper who will let you in when
your driver blows the car horn, and the compound is enclosed by a tall brick or stone wall,
often with broken glass or barbed wire on top
of this wall. Dogs are usually let out to roam

the compound at night. Years ago, I stayed at one compound in Kenya where there was a guard who roamed the grounds at night with a bow and arrow. With all of this protection, you will be quite safe.

Food & Drink

Food is simple, and you will probably eat the same thing every day. Many African countries eat a form of corn flour and water, made into a "porridge" that is relatively tasteless and eaten with their hands (along with most other foods). This food is called "ugali" in Kenya, "nshima" in Zambia; it is eaten once or twice a day, every day, and it looks similar to mashed potatoes. Try it, you might even enjoy it.

It is a common practice to always wash your hands before eating - even in restaurants, there will be a sink. If you are at someone's home, a girl may come around with a pitcher of water and a basin, maybe some soap, and a towel. Put your hands out and allow her to pour the water over your hands as you rub them together to wash over the basin, then take the towel she hands you to dry your hands, and allow her to move on to the rest of the people present.

When in Africa, do like the Africans. Alcohol is generally forbidden among "respectable" people, so do not drink any alcohol while in your visiting country, or you may be disrespected. You will probably drink a lot of tea, which is more frequently consumed than coffee since it is much cheaper. Don't forget – do not drink the water or brush your teeth with the water. Purchase bottled water from stores, never on the street, *and do not drink the water if the seal is broken.* Remember, do not buy food from the street markets - ask to be driven to town for your drinking water and any supplies or food you may need.

Money

When packing any cash before you leave America, separate your money and place it in various locations in case you lose an item or have anything stolen. It is safest to use debit and/or credit cards so you do not have to carry much cash. When exchanging money, you always lose some value, so exchange only what you need, and do not exchange all of your money until you know what your expenses are and how much of the local currency you will actually need. Money can be confusing at first, until you learn the exchange rate of the currency. Go with one of your African friends to a bank or bureau (or if there is an exchange at the airport) and look for the best rate to exchange your money, preferably with no commission fees.

When shopping, have an African friend with you as well, since you may not understand the currency and may not pay the correct amount, or you may not get back the correct change if you appear unsure. Also, bargaining occurs at all the street markets/ shops, and you will be told higher prices than normal if you look like you are not from the country you are visiting – especially if you are a white American; you will automatically be assumed to be rich, and in comparison to most of the people there, you are. Usually the price you will be quoted is double of the actual price, so go with African friends to prevent financial difficulties.

Communication

If you are in a rural area, most of the patients may not speak English, though the hospice staff will. However, we can still communicate with others through smiles and touch. Africans always shake hands, so be ready to shake hands each time you greet someone. I prayed with people who did not speak English, but I was able to communicate enough to ask if they wanted prayer, and if they did, we prayed together – the patient in their language, and I prayed in English. It was beautiful. You can also ask one of your hospice workers to translate for a conversation as well.

Internet access is quite problematic, and you may not be able to communicate with friends, family and work. Hopefully, your hospice will allow you to use their service (when it is running), and at least be able to inform people back home that you are safe and busy.

Church

Many Africans are very "religious" and spend a lot of time in church, so be prepared to attend on Sunday, possibly all day. Church almost always lasts more than an hour. I attended one church in a small rural village that lasted from 5:00 a.m. until 1:00 pm, though we arrived late (of course). Most churches do not last that long, but they often worship for a few hours in the morning, have a meal, and come back together in the afternoon.

If you are a chaplain or pastor, be prepared to preach at church on Sunday if you attend a Protestant church; come with a sermon or two. If you are not a chaplain or pastor, at least be prepared to go to church and to be brought up to the front of the congregation to bring greetings from America and to say a few words. If possible, use the local language for a few words.

When you are feeling only your losses,
then everything around you speaks of them.
The trees, the flowers, the clouds, the hills
and valleys, they all reflect your sadness.

Henri Nouwen

Chapter Three

Processing Emotions

It was not until my second trip to Africa that I was able to see past the suffering, to the beauty and hope that continues to exist in the midst of unbelievable poverty. There is "another Africa" where I saw past the poverty, the mud, the noise and the chaos, to the beauty of the land, the varied and abundant wild life, and the people who do not live such desperate lives.

If this will be your first trip to a Third World country, the poverty may overwhelm you and you may find yourself becoming depressed. The first time I went to Africa (Kenya), I was unable to see the beauty of the land because the poverty I saw clouded everything else. Many parts of Africa are indeed very poor, with abject poverty such as you have probably never seen or experienced.

If you have the time and money, I urge you to get away for a few days for several reasons. Living in Third World poverty is quite overwhelming and depressing; before heading back to the States, you may want to process your emotions, away from the poverty. There are some beautiful areas in probably all of the

African countries, and no trip to Africa is complete without a safari.

When in Africa, you may have many HIV positive patients, who are also quite young. Your emotions will need a reprieve from the sadness, the poverty, and the feelings of helplessness that may have crept into your soul. Getting away for at least a couple of days brings a more balanced view of Africa, and prepares you for your long journey back home. As in all hospice work, there is a need for a healthy balance.

In Zambia, I visited Victoria Falls, which were amazingly beautiful, and which are one of the Seven Wonders of the World. I also went on an elephant back safari, interacted with lions, and canoed the great Zambezi River. I had a great time. There are many affordable lodges and tented camps where you can stay that usually include a full breakfast. Even if you get away for only one night before heading home, it is beneficial, though if you can get away for several nights, it would be a good idea. I have traveled many times to Kenya in the past (for non-hospice related work), and all of my missionary friends suggest this same idea of getting away in order to process your emotions and gain a balanced view of Africa.

Keep in mind though, that most, if not all of the people from the hospice have probably not gone to the places you may wish to visit, so do so on your way home, perhaps not even mentioning it. At least, keep the "vacation" talk to a minimum. Inform your African hospice colleagues of any financial help you received to make the trip possible, and that this "vacation" is primarily your desire to see the beauty of their country. Be sensitive.

You may want to keep a journal of your trip. Your emotions might be all over the place, and it is healthy to write them down, especially if you are traveling alone. If you are with others, get together in the evenings and share your thoughts. Living together for a while in Africa might also be a good place to brainstorm fund-raising ideas and other creative ways to assist your partnered hospice. Being with other people away from the poverty-stricken hospice, having fun together, and sharing life-long memories are healthy and meaningful.

What have you learned since seeing an African hospice and the conditions in which they operate? What are the cultural considerations you are now beginning to observe, and how will these differences affect how you partner in the future with an African hospice? How are you and your partner different? How are you the same? What things do you need to be more sensitive about? What is the best way to assist your hospice partner? What have you learned about the people with whom you have interacted? What have they taught you?

These questions are just a few ideas for processing your thoughts, which you will need to do before heading home, while they are still fresh in your mind, and your excitement, enthusiasm, and love for your new friends is still vibrant.

Most Americans develop a different perspective on life after traveling to Third World countries. The things many Americans consider "necessary" might now appear as luxuries, and hopefully you will appreciate the things you have far more than before you traveled. Many of us look at our kitchens and bathrooms and decide they "need" to be updated – until you see an outdoor kitchen and bathroom made of mud or sticks and plastic.

Hopefully, you will understand just how blessed we truly are. Do you have a job? Do you have a car? Do you have a bank account? Do you eat every day? Do you have heat/air conditioning? Do you have indoor plumbing? Do you enjoy any luxuries, such as traveling to Africa? If you lost your job, would you be able to collect unemployment? Do you have any savings to rely on when finances become difficult? Is there a food pantry at any of the local churches or community centers in your neighborhood? Can you collect disability if you were unable to work? Is there government assistance to rely on if the need arose?

Many countries do not have these American safety nets, and surely the country you visit in Africa does not. People rely on family, friends, and God. If you can say "yes" to any of the above questions, then you are in the minority of people on this earth; most people do not live the way Americans do, but more like the people you will see or have seen in your African country. While many complain about different things in America, we are indeed very blessed.

Remember that all mission work is a two-way path of learning and growing. As the American hospices, we go to deepen our relationships with the poor African hospices, to assess needs, and to discover how their hospices function in order to form the most beneficial partnership possible. We can share our knowledge with them, and they in turn can share their knowledge and insights with us. The late Priest and author, Henri Nouwen, wrote a beautiful summary about overseas mission work, though I believe his ideas apply here as well, concerning hospice work. While Nouwen wrote about sharing the message of Jesus with others, we can take his same principle within our work and translate the ideas into sharing our "mission" of hospice and palliative care work, as well as the love and compassion of Jesus. As a chaplain, I find the following quote especially beautiful. Nouwen wrote:

*"Here we realize that missions is not only
to go and tell others about the risen Lord, but
also to receive that witness from those to whom
we are sent. Often, mission is thought of ex-
clusively in terms of giving, but true mission
is also receiving. If it is true that the Spirit of
Jesus blows where it wants, there is no person
who cannot give that spirit. In the long run,
mission is only possible when it is as much
receiving as giving, as much being cared for as
caring. We are sent to the sick, the dying, the
handicapped...We will soon be burned out if we
cannot receive the spirit of the Lord from those
to whom we are sent. Each time we reach out,
they in turn, whether they are aware or not,
will bless us with the Spirit of Jesus and so
become our ministers. Without this mutuality of
giving and receiving, mission and ministry eas-
ily become manipulative and violent. When only
one gives and the other receives, the giver will
soon become the oppressor, and the receivers,
victims. But when the giver receives and the re-
ceiver gives, the circle of love can grow as wide
as the world"* (Nouwen, 1994, p.115-116).

"We can do no great things;
only small things with great love."

Mother Teresa

At the end of our life, we shall be judged by love.

Saint John of the Cross

Chapter Four

Getting Involved

Some Americans say, "We have needs here in our own country; why should we help Africa? Shouldn't we help our own people first? Our hospice here in America has needs too!" While these statements are true, the need is so great and the resources are simply not available in Africa as they are in America.

The hospice in Zambia received very little government funding, there was no Medicare or Medicaid plan, no private insurance plans to cover hospice services, and even the staff salaries were paid by a grant that was coming to an end. I asked the staff what they are doing to ensure their salaries continue to be paid, and they replied that they are researching other grants, trying to get more people involved, including the Zambian government, and praying a lot. This Zambian hospice was truly faith-based and a missional hospice.

The funding for the particular hospice that I visited in Zambia came from Catholic Relief Services, founder churches, including the Lutheran Church, local service clubs, local communities, the District Health Management Team through the Zambian government, and

DAFA (Direct Aid for Africa). They also receive grants, for specific periods of time from Catholic Relief Services, Princes Diana Memorial Fund of Wales, and Irish Aid through Buyantashi Ecumenical Women's Group.

Catholic Relief Services provides the majority of funding for this hospice by helping with food, prescription drugs, cleaning materials, staff training, office equipment, repairs and maintenance of their buildings. The churches in Africa appear to understand the importance of end of life care, and are the founders and primary sustainers of many hospices. Sadly, the American church and missionaries have little involvement in end of life care.

The caregivers in Zambia, who are similar to our American nurse aides, worked for years for free, because they loved the work and felt they needed to give back to the communities where they lived, and they wanted to serve God in this manner. Some of the caregivers told me that they believe God has forgiven them from their past mistakes, and they want to help others deal with possibly some of their own mistakes in a loving and forgiving manner. Finally, they are now paid, though very little, and most of the caregivers live in the extremely poor compounds in mud homes, such as I visited with the nurses when we did the home-based care.

The manager of the hospice I visited in Zambia told me that they have occasionally found dying people lying at the gate of their hospice when they arrived for work. When a poor family realizes their loved one is dying, and they have no money to care for that person or to pay for their loved ones final expenses, they sometimes leave their family member at the entrance of the hospice. This is done because they know the hospice workers will take that person inside, give them a clean bed, feed them, and care for them until death. Consequently, the hospice has been forced to bury the dead themselves, since in situations like these, they have no one to contact. Can you imagine leaving your dying parent, spouse, child, or any other loved one alone on the street at night, waiting for a hospice worker to carry that person inside? This is the harsh reality of many parts of Africa, and that is why Christians should be involved in missional hospice care; to show that they care.

Hospice and palliative care has to be rationed in Zambia, since they do not have the money to provide end of life care to all people in need. Compassionate hospice care is only available to the poorest of the poor, since the hospice workers hope other sick and dying people in Zambia, who are *not* among the most poor, can afford to have people (though untrained) care for them at the end of life. In America, all people are entitled to hospice and palliative care; one's socio-economic status is not a factor, nor does it prohibit anyone from receiving such care. Americans need to share their many blessings with Africans who do not have access to compassionate, trained, quality care as we have for people at their most crucial and often most desperate and painful time of life – the end of life.

If you have the passion to go to Africa as a hospice worker or as a missionary, I pray that you have a blessed and fruitful visit. Hopefully, you will make wonderful new friends, and share your passion for people. In helping the vulnerable, the sick, and the dying, I hope you will feel as much love from your African friends as I have felt and continue to feel from mine.

Here are just a couple (of the many) verses in the Bible that speak about our responsibilities to the poor:

God Multiplies the Seed Sown

9. As it is written, his generosity is scattered to the poor; his love-deeds are never forgotten. 10. Now he who supplies plenty of seed for the planting also furnishes bread for your table, and multiplies the seed sown and increases the fruit of your benevolence; (2 Corinthians 9:9, 10 EDNT)

Practice Generosity to all

9. And let us not become weary in doing what is right: for if we do not weaken our resolve, in due season we will collect the good harvest. 10. As we have opportunity, let us practice generosity to all. (Galatians 6:9 -10a EDNT)

Let us touch
the dying, the poor, the lonely and the unwanted
according to the graces we have received,
and let us not be ashamed or slow
to do the humble work.

Mother Teresa

Chapter Five

Undertaking a Missional Hospice

What is a missionary? Webster's Dictionary defines a missionary simply as, "a person undertaking a mission." As a chaplain, when talking to many people at the end of their lives, they often reflect on what was the meaning and purpose of their lives; in other words, what mission did they undertake in the time they were given? Have you thought about your own undertaking in life? What might be your mission? People who work in hospice generally understand their mission to be caring for people at the end of life; specifically, hospice chaplains define their mission as caring for people's spiritual well-being at the end of life.

When we think of missionaries, Americans often think of someone going to Africa to help the poor and share the Gospel through teaching, preaching and planting churches. Life is busy and hectic for us all, and we of course concentrate on providing daily needs and on living, which traditionally is also the focus of missionaries. But might some missionaries focus on the dying, and the many needs that are present at that time of life, which can be addressed through hospice work? Missionaries work in various types of settings, such as in medical missions, preaching, teaching, church planting, children's ministries, feeding centers, pilots, immediate relief work in times of natural disasters, construction work, etc. Consider hospice work in a missional context as well, which includes several of the already traditional forms of missionary work, but also, like Mother Teresa's home for the dying, a focus on the inevitable for us all – death, and the multitude of difficulties, grief and pain it brings to us all, and in making that transition more comfortable, both physically and spiritually.

Mother Teresa fought hard to establish compassionate end of life care in Calcutta India, which is done under the supervision and blessing of the Catholic Church, and carried out by the Missionaries of Charity. While the Home for the Dying is attached to the Hindu Temple, Kalighad, Mother Teresa's hospice is unashamedly Christian. This hospice was begun by the Catholic Church, who understands the crucial need for end of life care. In her book, *"No Greater Love,"* Mother Teresa recounted a story of a dying woman the Missionaries of Charity picked up off the streets. Mother Teresa wrote:

"In twenty-five years, we have picked up more than thirty-six thousand people from the

streets and more than eighteen thousand have died a most beautiful death. When we pick them up from the street we give them a plate of rice. In no time we revive them. A few nights ago we picked up four people. One was in a most terrible condition, covered with wounds, full of maggots. I told the sisters that I would take care of her while they attended to the other three. I really did all that my love could do for her. I put her in bed and then she took hold of my hand. She had such a beautiful smile on her face and said only, 'Thank you.' Then she died.

There was a greatness of love. She was hungry for love, and she received that love before she died. She spoke only two words, but her understanding love was expressed in those two words." (Mother Teresa, *No Greater Love*, (1997,137-138).

I was privileged a few years ago to go to Calcutta, India and work at Mother Teresa's home for the dying, and witness stories such as the one you just read. The Missionaries of Charity have also opened such homes for the dying throughout the United States, often with a focus on AIDS patients. Does Mother Teresa's story sound much different from the hospice manager's story in Zambia about finding poor, dying people lying alone at their hospice compound's gate? How can the American churches not be impacted by these stories? Why does the Catholic Church support such important work, but many Protestant churches, of which I am a member, do not? I have yet to hear of a Protestant missionary going to Africa to work primarily with a hospice, or with dying people, living on the threshold of eternity, yet the needs and the challenges are so great.

In Zambia, the hospice I worked with spoke of the many challenges that we do not encounter in America, such as inadequate funding to provide the highest possible care to their patients, and therefore must implement inadequately trained personnel. In job interviews at American hospices, all disciplines must be adequately trained: chaplains must hold Masters of Divinity degrees, Clinical Pastoral Education, ordination and Ecclesiastical endorsements; social workers usually require Masters Degrees; nurses must have their nursing educations and licenses, and nurse aids are also trained and certified. No one in any of these disciplines would even be granted an interview without the proper credentials; this is not the case in Africa.

Also, hospice and palliative care is a new concept in Africa, and the need is great to have qualified, trained, educated people to assist those in need who are suffering and dying. Another aspect of care in African hospices, which Americans have no need to even consider, is kitchen and laundry equipment, which we take for granted. Electricity is scarce in rural Africa, and the ability to maintain clean bedding for patients and sanitary meal preparation is quite challenging. People who are sick and/or incontinent obviously need frequent changes of clean bedding which is difficult in rural Africa, since most laundry is washed by hand and hung out to dry. Also, healthy, adequate food is often a problem due to lack of funding, and patients who are HIV positive need a healthy diet or their medications will be of no value.

We all of course will someday die. People of faith believe we will all face God at that time, so why would a missionary not be concerned for people's spiritual well-being while preparing for their death, and for their soul in eternity? Surely hospice work can, and should indeed be missionary work as well.

"At the moment of death, we will not be judged by the amount of work we have done but by the weight of love we have put into our work. This love should flow from self-sacrifice, and it must be felt to the point of hurting. Death, in the final analysis, is only the easiest and quickest means to go back to God. If only we could make people understand that we come from God and that we have to go back to Him! Death is the most decisive moment in human life. It is our coronation: to die in peace with God." (Mother Teresa: No Greater Love (1997, 140-141).

*It is only the broken soil that can receive the water
and make the seed grow and bear fruit.*

Henri Nouwen

Chapter Six

Turning Over a Few Stones

Your presence in Africa can make a difference. You may not realize the impact of your visit to Africa, but you and God together clearly contribute to changing things for the better. Something as simple as turning over a stone can speak volumes, "I was here. I care about you. I am aware of your needs." When I first read the book "*Turning Stones*," it was not clear what the author meant. Near the end of Marc Parent's book, he wrote about a nun traveling in remote places who turned over stones as she went. Someone asked why she turned over stones, and her response opened my eyes. She explained that turning over a stone was a tangible way to say something is different because she was here. I think about her response often. Should not places and people be different because we were there? It is never too late to turn over a stone in someone's life, even during the end of life struggles. Turning over a few stones so others may see the other side of an issue is an important function of a missional traveler.

You may feel that you left everything comfortable, familiar, easy and orderly when you arrived in rural Africa. It may have felt like another world that you have never experienced before. Africa is vastly different from America in many ways. The pharmacist at the hospice I visited in Zambia is from England, though she has now lived in Zambia for about thirty years. She said when people in Europe ask her how Africa compares to England, she tells them she felt like she was dropped off on another planet. There is no comparison. However, you may have noticed that despite cultural differences, all people are generally the same; we all have hopes and dreams, we all have desires, thoughts and emotions – we just live them out in different settings. All people are created in God's image, and are all part of one race, the human race, whose beauty lies in cultural differences and mutual understandings.

Returning to America

Hopefully, you have made some wonderful new friends, which will last for many years. You now have a clearer picture of how you can strengthen your partnership. Your heart will probably be broken by much that you have seen and experienced, but as Henri Nouwen suggested, personal and spiritual growth will be the result of that brokenness. "It is only the broken soil that can receive the water and make the seed grow and bear fruit."

You will take away from Africa many rich memories, and leave behind many fond memories, love, friendship, and perhaps something tangible. If you are able, you may leave behind a cash donation or some type of gift, especially if you have been accommodated for free, in order to express tangibly your gratitude and appreciation. If you stay in someone's home, be sure to leave a gift for their hospitality. I have found that the people who have the least always give the most. Be prepared to receive gifts when you leave. Each time I have left an African country, I have been given gifts. The day before I was to leave Zambia, I was "called into the office," unsure of what I had done wrong. I was then showered with many beautiful gifts. I was so overwhelmed, I was brought to tears. The following day (the day of my departure), I was given even more gifts, and everyone came to my guest house to say goodbye. I was deeply touched. Be prepared for tearful good-byes when you depart.

Bringing a few souvenirs and keepsakes from Africa to America may solidify your desire to utilize the compassion you felt there to enhance your work and mission back home. These tokens of your visit become reminders of what you experienced. Now the real work of missional hospice begins. Having seen the pain and poverty in parts of Africa, you are in a better position to make a difference in your patient's care at home. You can convert the compassion developed more fully in Africa, to intensify your patient care in the American end of life system.

There may be no comparison between Africa and America, but there is common ground when the missional concept of hospice is remembered. Those involved in hospice are involved because they care about people and understand the end of life needs for terminal patients. People under hospice care have special needs that include medical, psychological, personal, relational, spiritual, and eternal concerns. Hospice workers do not only manage physical pain and make patients comfortable, but they assist their concerns regarding after their death, whatever their faith or religion. These concerns must be addressed in a missional approach to hospice.

About the Author

Donna Kasik is a native of the Chicago suburbs where she lived until her mid-forties. She owned her own business as a painter in the construction trades while attending college and seminary at night for many years. After earning an under-graduate degree in Philosophy and a Masters of Divinity, she left the Chicago-land area for Kentucky and other states as she completed her Clinical Pastoral Education.

Ms. Kasik is ordained through the Evangelical Church Alliance. Her passion though, is cultural studies and mission work. She taught at a seminary in Kenya, East Africa, for 6 years, short-term intensives each of those years, worked at Mother Teresa's home for the dying in Calcutta, India, and worked at an AIDS hospice in Zambia, Africa.

A Hospice Chaplain in Kentucky, the author will begin a Doctor of Ministry in Missional Leadership in 2013, for continued learning in cultural studies and of sharing her faith in various cultures. Donna loves to travel, read, write, cook, run, the Arts, and all outdoor activities. She is active in her local church and community, and serves in her Ministerial Association.

Donna has one son, of whom she is very proud, and she expresses gratitude for a wonderful daughter-in-law. A source of delight is her new granddaughter and step-grandson. The greatest joy in life for Donna is being a follower of Jesus Christ, who brings peace that passes understanding, along with joy and contentment that the world could never give.

~

Other Books by the Author

Kenya: A Priority on My Bucket List
ISBN: 978-1-935434-63-4

Recovery: A Return to the Self
ISBN: 978-1-935434-51-1

Thinking Outside the Box ...About Love
ISBN: 978-1-935434-00-5

Order books from the Global Bookstore:

www.gea-books.com/bookstore/browse by author/

References

Green, Hollis L. (Translator) (2012) *The Evergreen Devotional New Testament (EDNT).* Complete Edition, Post-Gutenberg Books: GlobalEdAdvance Press.

Kasik, Donna. (2009) *Thinking Outside the Box...About Love.* Nashville, GlobalEdAdvance Press.

Kasik, Donna. (2010) *Recovery: A Return to the Self.* Nashville, GlobalEdAdvance Press.

Kasik, Donna. (2012) *KENYA: A Priority on my Bucket List.* Nashville, GlobalEdAdvance Press.

Mother Teresa. (1997) *No Greater Love.* New World Library, Novato, California.

Nouwen, Henri J.M. (1994)*With Burning Hearts: A Meditation on the Eucharistic Life.* Orbis Books, Maryknoll, New York.

Parent, Marc. (1996) *Turning Stones: My Days and Nights with Children at Risk.* New York: Harcourt Brace and Company.

Stetzer, Ed, Putman, David. (2006) *Breaking the Missional Code: Your Church can become a Missionary in your Community.* Nashville: Broadman & Holman.

www.ingramcontent.com/pod-product-compliance
Lightning Source LLC
Chambersburg PA
CBHW031527040426
42445CB00009B/432